NATURAL ROSACEA TREATMENT

How to Reduce Inflammation in the Skin, Balance the body and Control Face and Scalp Seborrheic Dermatitis, Dandruff and Psoriasis Problems at Any Age.

By Ori Laor

Disclaimer

The methods described within this eBook are the author's personal thoughts. They are not intended to be a definitive set of instructions for this project. You may discover there are other methods and materials to accomplish the same end result.

This book is not intended to be a substitute for the medical advice of a licensed physician. The reader should consult with their doctor in any matters relating to his/her health.

Before beginning any new exercise program, it is recommended that you seek medical advice from your personal physician.

The information contained within this eBook is strictly for educational purposes. If you wish to apply ideas contained in this eBook, you are taking full responsibility for your actions.

The author has made every effort to ensure the accuracy of the information within this book was correct at time of publication. The author does not assume and hereby disclaims any liability to any party for any loss, damage, or disruption caused by errors or omissions, whether such errors or omissions result from accident, negligence, or any other cause.

Thank you very much
Ori Laor

Table of Contents

Personal Introduction

Thank you for downloading this fantastic guide- "Natural Rosacea Treatment." This book will provide you with all the information I have obtained up to date about clearing skin disorders. Has an Aesthetician I have treated many people with Rosacea, Seborrheic dermatitis, Eczema, and psoriasis over the last 20 years. It is my hope that the knowledge contained within this book can help you overcome your skin condition and live life to your fullest potential, You can always feel free to contact me for more clarifications.

Rosacea or Seborrheic dermatitis is a common skin condition seen frequently in clinical practice. The use of varying terms such as Sebo psoriasis, seborrheic dermatitis, seborrheic eczema, dandruff, and pityriasis capitis reflects the complex nature of this condition.

If you've noticed scaly patches on your face or body, you could be experiencing seborrheic dermatitis. This is a common, inflammatory skin condition involving a rash, usually pink in color, and areas of scaling that are typically white or yellow. Although unrelated, seborrheic dermatitis has been known to occur at the same time as rosacea.The rash may or may not be itchy, but mostly seborrheic dermatitis is disfiguring and just really disturbing. If you can see symptoms on your scalp, this is referred to as dandruff.

The causes of Rosacea and seborrheic dermatitis are relatively unknown at this stage, but there are several working theories which by the end of this page, we hope you will obtain the necessary information required to help you solve seborrheic challenges.

We hope these resources will prove useful to the widest possible audience seeking information on Rosacea and seborrheic dermatitis.

For my new Creatspace and Kindle readers, I offer a Free Voucher Gift of 20$. You can find a keyword at the end of this book. Please send it to my mail orilaor@outlook.com, and you will receive a discount for any porches you make for yourself, a member of your family or a friend in LAOR website www.laorcare.com.

About Me

I have a passion for Beauty, Skincare, Anti-aging and well-being methods. In my extensive exploration around the world, I gathered sacred pieces of information that helped me and then other people from all walks of life to look and feel younger. I hold a BA in Art and diplomas for Makeup Artist, Para Medical Aesthetician, Aromatherapy, Naturopathy, and Nutrition consultant. I am a well-known name in T.V scene and in the cosmetic industry, including treating many celebrities. When I was 30 years old, I quit working for others and founded LAOR, a House of natural Beauty and Professional Skin Care and treatments for the face, Body, and Mind.

Since an early age, I suffered from my skin and was carried away with Skincare research, science and well-being. I worked in beauty and style departments in New York and Tel Aviv, based on my experience I invented a revolutionary practice for treating the skin from within – **The Layer system**, Complied with a line of professional cosmetic products and treatments for the face to treat any skin problem.

Ientered the natural cosmetics world with a unique world-view and with one simple, honest purpose: to create a different kind of cosmetic that is Natural and effective. My desire is that each product would provide each with the essence of beauty, based on effective ingredients.

Now, for the past Two Decades, I am designing the products that Men and women across the world love, helping them to look and feel younger with all the secrets of skin care. When I am not working, I love to design and create, read, write and paint. My quest is to bring more beauty to the world and raise self-awareness.

Let's Get Started!

Chapter 1

Skin Disorders

The Reasons

If you are reading this book you probably have some skin disorder like disturbing greasy skin, scaly rashes and dryness on your face, eyebrows, nose, ears, chin, chest or scalp and they appear red and sometimes looks like pimples. You may have something called seborrheic dermatitis better known as Rosacea and dandruff. In babies, it is commonly referred to as "cradle cap."

Seborrhea is a common skin problem. It causes a red, itchy rash and white scales. When it affects the scalp, it is called "dandruff." It can be on parts of the face as well, including the folds around the nose and behind the ears, the forehead, and the eyebrows and eyelids. On the body, seborrhea often occurs in the middle part of the chest, around the navel and in the skin folds under the arm, below the breasts and in the groin and buttocks area.

This is a widespread condition that I see on a daily basis. It can be very challenging to have as well as tricky to treat. So often patients try to figure out what is wrong with their skin and are frustrated after trying almost any skin care available that does not work.

Seborrheic dermatitis is absolutely not due to a lack of hygiene! Scalp dandruff is not a result of not washing your hair frequently enough. It's also not due to a dry scalp from washing your hair too often! The exact cause of this issue can be complicated, as you will see later in this book. However, it is essential to know that you may not be able to treat your seborrheic dermatitis on your own.

The cause of this skin problem is not completely understood, but we do know that it is associated with overgrowth of yeast (fungus) called Malassezia that is in oil-secreting areas of our skin. This leads to inflammation, scale and sometimes swelling of the skin from the inflammatory reaction Malassezia causes.

Seborrheic dermatitis overlaps with two conditions. The most common overlap I see is with rosacea. People may have a combination of any rosacea subtype and seborrheic dermatitis.

The second most common skin problem I see in combination with seborrheic dermatitis is psoriasis. When these two conditions overlap, it is called "Sebo-psoriasis."

It's actually imperative to moisturize your skin when you have seborrheic dermatitis not only to soften those skin flakes but also to soothe your skin that is inflamed. One way of soothing the skin is by using a topical steroid, which you can buy over the counter or get a prescription from your doctor, but Be careful, this creams harms the skin and make it thin and week over time also they lose the effect on the skin after some time and the problem comes back even worse, some prescription steroids should never be used on facial skin. Steroids calm inflammation but don't do much in the way of moisturizing the skin. I suggest that before jumping to using topical steroids, why not try a natural product that can calm and treat the skin with no risk for the long run.

When seborrheic dermatitis is very severe, it could actually be related to other internal causes. I keep certain medical problems in the back of my mind when I see stubborn, rampant cases of seborrheic dermatitis-like: Parkinson's Disease, Stroke, HIV, Alcoholism and Nutritional Disorders.

Rosacea, seborrheic dermatitis, psoriasis, and Dandruff are not contagious, so there is no way to prevent it. It's also not possible to "cure," but we can certainly control it with the measures I will describe in this book. These conditions of the skin that can be embarrassing, causing flakes of skin to appear in the face and hair and fall onto clothes. Dandruff is a common condition marked by itching, and in some cases is not easy to treat.There is a natural cycle of skin renewal that can be caused to speed up, leading to patches of dead skin forming on the surface of the scalp.

What causes the skin renewal cycle to speed up is not always clear, but below you will find the typical causes for skin disorders:

Seborrheic Dermatitis

This is a very common condition that causes oily skin, and people with it are very prone to dandruff. This can also affect many areas of the skin, including the backs of the ears, the breastbone, eyebrows, the sides of the nose and anywhere where skin folds together, such as the armpits. It causes red, greasy skin that's covered with flaky white or yellow scales.

These two issues are thought to be interlinked, as the presence of the fungus on skin may provoke an abnormal response from the immune system, which can then cause skin to become oily. Then, the oiliness of the skin, encourages more growth of the fungus, which then triggers dandruff.

Leaky Gut Syndrome

We can develop allergic reactions by having an already-weakened immune response or "leaky gut syndrome" (thinning and damaged small intestinal walls that leak toxins into the bloodstream). In a vicious cycle, allergens in our food or medications continue wearing away the gastrointestinal tract, allowing more and more toxicity and undigested protein molecules to circulate. Our body's natural response is to produce extra white blood cells, releasing more histamine; eventually inflammation develops as a safety mechanism.

Candida Growth and Probiotics

Probiotic usage has been extremely useful in the healing of Candida issues, which cause seborrheic dermatitis."Everyone's body is host to Candida. Candida is a type of yeast. Candida is normally kept under control by good health and probiotics. However, Candida overgrowth can occur when the system is challenged or altered. The use of antibiotics can reduce the ability of probiotics to keep Candida at bay. Also, the over-consumption of yeast-feeding foods such as simple carbohydrates, sugars, peanuts, alcohol and milk products can encourage Candida growth.

Seborrheic dermatitis is a skin condition. The skin cells are directly connected with the large intestine, therefore problems with the skin are linked to digestion, issues with stomach acids and gut imbalances. Children exhibiting this skin disorder do well to eat greater amounts of fruits and vegetables, while eliminating the major allergenic foods. Children who spend time outdoors in the sunshine and sleep in well-ventilated rooms also experience improvement.

Fungus (Malassezia)

Malassezia is a fungus that lives on everybody's scalp, and typically causes no issues at all, but it can grow out of control. It feeds on the oils our hair follicles secrete, then causes the scalp can become irritated and produce other skin cells. These extra skin cells die and fall off, then mixes with the oil on the hair and scalp. Reddish, scaly plaques may also appear in the eyebrows, on the forehead, in the ear canal, on the folds of skin that extend from the nostril to the lips. Although the skin affected may feel and look dry, this is not the case.

Yeast

People who are sensitive to yeast have a slightly higher risk of having dandruff and other skin disorders. These yeast-sensitive people find that it gets better during the warmer months and worse during the winter. UVA light from the sun counteracts the yeast. The skin is drier due to cold air and overheated rooms during the winter, making dandruff more likely. So, it is sometimes not that easy to know whether it is yeast or just dry skin.

Dandruff

People with psoriasis, eczema, and other skin disorders tend to get dandruff much more frequently than other people. Other conditions like the cold winter air, combined with overheated rooms is a common cause of dandruff because of it creates dry skin that presents itself as small flakes of dandruff, that are not oily.

In Babies

Babies wear diapers most of the time. This gives rise to moist skin for long hours of the day which crinkles their skin and exposes them to germs and bacteria. This can be the cause of flaky and irritable skin, accompanied by rashes and red patches. This condition is also very common on the scalp of babies. Although it subsides over the initial growing period, the redness, itching and patches on the scalp are ugly and uncomfortable to deal with.

In Adults

Seborreic Dermatitis in adults mainly results from dry skin, yeast infection, allergies and bad eating habits. Sometimes people lack the natural oil that is produced by their skin on a daily basis. This dries skin up excessively. We all have the yeast Malassezia furfur in our bodies. However, those who have this yeast in large doses are more prone to Seborrheic Dermatitis.

A lot of people confuse Seborreic Dermatitis with dandruff because this affects the scalp as well. However, this is different from dandruff. It is a disease that generates from allergies and skin conditions. Dandruff on the other hand is the result of bad lifestyle.

The Causes

The exact cause of Rosacea and seborrheic dermatitis is unknown. Doctors thinks it may be due to a combination hormone levels, weakened immune system, lack of certain nutrients, or nervous system problems. Irritation from a yeast called Malassezia may also lead to this condition. Seborrheic dermatitis appears to run in families, This factors include:

- Stress or fatigue

- Weather extremes

- Oily skin, or skin problems such as acne

- Infrequent shampoos or skin cleaning

- Using lotions that contain alcohol, chemicals, and mineral oil

- Obesity

- Neurologic conditions, including Parkinson's disease, head injury or stroke

- Human immunodeficiency virus (HIV)

Symptoms

Seborrheic dermatitis can occur on different body areas. Usually it forms where the skin is oily or greasy. Common areas include the scalp, eyebrows, eyelids, creases of the nose, lips, behind the ears, in the outer ear, and middle of the chest. So how do you know you have seborrheic dermatitis and not something else? Well, the easiest way to tell is if you have a combination of the following symptoms:

- Dryness

- Hair loss

- Patches of greasy skin covered with skin flakes

- Patches of white or yellow scales

- Redness and irritation - may become more itchy if infected

- Itching, burning and crawling sensation of the skin

- On the scalp, it is most commonly referred to simply as dandruff. On the face, however, it almost always goes by the name of seborrheic dermatitis. Essentially, they are the same thing.

When seborrheic dermatitis occurs elsewhere than the scalp, it also looks visually similar to eczema. These two conditions are quite similar in nature, and the biggest difference appears to be the greasiness and scaling that accompanies seborrheic dermatitis. Eczema typically has dryer crusting and less flaking.

Commonly Affected Areas

The most common areas for seborrheic dermatitis are the scalp, nasal folds, ears and other hair-bearing areas of the face. For the most part, people believe that this is due to these areas having the most sebaceous activity (sweat and oil production). Treating seborrheic dermatitis on the scalp (dandruff) is the most straight-forward and widely available dandruff shampoos can quickly produce good results for the short term. However, treating seborrheic dermatitis on the face can often pose a variety of difficulties due to the sensitive nature of the facial skin.

Why These Areas

The most common explanation is that seborrheic dermatitis occurs in these areas because of the heightened sebaceous activity mentioned above. However, I believe it is not as straightforward as that. Specifically, there are study that used thermal imagery to examine other possible factors affecting the location of seborrheic dermatitis. This study concluded that seborrheic dermatitis most commonly affected the warmer areas of the facial skin (source). This heightened facial temperature is likely responsible for attracting a greater amount of the bacteria present on the skin surface. As more bacteria accumulate in these warmer patches of skin, the seborrheic dermatitis can become triggered.

Prior to seeing the thermal images of the face, I had a hard time understanding why my seborrheic dermatitis often took the butterfly pattern. However, after seeing the images (source), everything made much more sense. Additionally, you can specifically see that the nasal folds and the inside of the eye sockets appear to be the warmest, and these are areas where people seem to have most difficulty.

Treatment

Medical Approach

Typically, most doctors will tell you that it is a lifelong condition influenced by genetics. They will also tell you that the best way to treat it are proper management. When they refer to managing seborrheic dermatitis, they typically imply one of three things: an anti-fungal solution, a antibiotic solution (if they are less familiar with seborrheic dermatitis), or a corticosteroid. These are all typically prescribed for a period of two weeks. But if the seborrheic dermatitis returns, then treatment is usually recommended on a long term basis.

Additionally, from my personal experience and from communication with others, it appears that most medical professionals provide patients with very little information on seborrheic dermatitis. Plus it seems that the recommended solution that the doctor will usually recommend depends on their own knowledge of the condition. The more up-to-date doctors seem to prescribe anti-fungals, while the less up-to-date simply go with a broad-spectrum antibiotic and corticosteroid cream.

Traditional Treatments

Topical treatments are the most commonly recommended solution for seborrheic dermatitis outbreaks. These include creams and shampoos that contain corticosteroids or hydrocortisone. But these methods of treatment can cause thinning of your skin over time. So, they can only be used for few weeks. Supplementing these treatments with an alternative or natural treatment can help decrease side effects over the long term.

Antibacterial gels are prescribed to certain people whose Seborrheic dermatitis is triggered by bacteria on the scalp. Metronidazole is the most common active ingredient in these gels. Antifungal shampoos and creams are also sometimes suggested.

Some doctors use light therapy to treat seborrheic dermatitis. For this treatment, the doctor exposes the affected area of your scalp or skin to ultraviolet light. It helps soothe the skin and reduce itching and redness.

When to see your doctor

See your doctor to talk about your symptoms and make sure that you are diagnosed correctly. If you've tried self-treating your Seborrheic dermatitis without success, it's possible that you need a different diagnosis. If your flare-ups become a constant presence in your life, or if you also have other symptoms. Your primary care physician will most likely refer you to a dermatologist. This skin doctor may want to run some tests and talk to you about other treatments.

Holistic Approach

The actual meaning of the word holistic health is defined as the "treatment of the whole person, and not just the issue." Inline with this definition, the holistic practitioners will focus on the overall health of the person first and then focus on specific answer to Rosacea and seborrheic dermatitis. Most of the items on their list can typically overlap with practically every other healthcondition. Purifying the body usually eliminate any skin disorder, so try first this steps before you go to a doctor:

- Avoid chlorine and fluoride in your water

- Avoid Dairy Products

- Reducing sodium intake

- Switching to natural products

- Eating whole, raw organic foods

- Cut sugar and simple carbohydrates

- Cut gluten all together

- Drink lots of water

- Get tested for "food intolerances."

- Avoid inflammatory foods

- Fix your Omega fat ratio

- Supplement with probiotics and enzymes

So, there you have it, the very core of all holistic advice. Additional items are further added to this list depending on the specific condition the patient describes. For seborrheic dermatitis, the things that are mentioned most often are Apple Cider Vinegar, Coconut Oil, Sea Salt and Tea Tree Oil; I will describe this method in detail later in this book. However, you don't really need to be a professional to find out about these. The internet is full of success stories on each, and they are even discussed in detail on my website. Overall, though, the most common holistic understanding of seborrheic dermatitis seems to be that you have inflammation and immune issues inside your body, and in order to control these issues you must bring your body back to best health.

Chapter 2

Food Connection

Food Choices

Seborrheic dermatitis most commonly occurs on the scalp but can affect any area of the body with a large number of oil glands.This inflammatory condition can cause redness, flaking, itching, and lesions. But your food choices can influence inflammation, a major player in skin conditions such as this. Responses to changes in the diet can vary between individuals with the same health problem, and no guarantees exist that avoiding certain foods will influence your symptoms.

Inflammantory Fats

Our body uses fats to produce hormones involved in the inflammatory response. The Western diet is heavy on omega-6 fatty acids, which promote the production of pro-inflammatory chemicals, and is lacking in omega-3 fatty acids, which help fight inflammation. This imbalance likely contributes to the high incidence of inflammatory conditions in these societies, according to an article in the December 2002 issue of the "Journal of the American College of Nutrition." Oils particularly high in omega-6 fats include vegetable oils such as corn, sunflower, safflower, and soybean. Read the ingredients of packaged foods carefully since they are typically prepared with these oils. Fats found in animal foods and trans fats also contribute to inflammation.

Less Carbohydrates

A diet high in carbohydrates that produce large spikes in insulin can also promote inflammation. Nurse practitioner Marcelle Pick, writing for the site Women to Women, explains that high insulin levels cause the immune system to act as if it needs to fight off a harmful substance, leading to elevated levels of pro-inflammatory chemicals that normally alert infection-fighting white blood cells that they are needed. When no invader is actually present and inflammation is prolonged and constant, it can cause problems, such as inflammatory skin conditions. Problematic foods include processed carbohydrates such as white bread, soda and sugary foods such as cookies and candy. Carbohydrates that promote normal insulin levels include whole grains such as oatmeal and brown rice.

Your Diet

Dietary changes are most often successful because they address the root of the problem. The cause of seborrheic dermatitis and the cure of the condition are dependent on dietary and lifestyle changes. Eliminating refined sugars and white flour, which both feed yeasts, would be a first step. The second step is taking out all dairy products from the diet.

When trying to determine what their child is allergic to, parents often incorrectly assume that if he has eaten a food before and not had problems, then he probably is not allergic to that food. They usually only suspect new foods as being able to cause food allergies. However, it is important to keep in mind that it takes time for the immune system to build up a reaction against something that the body is allergic to. It may take days, weeks, months or even years to build up enough of a response to cause noticeable symptoms. So your child may be allergic to a food even if he has eaten it many times before, without problems.

A primary step should be to eliminate the main food challenges, as there is a strong proven link between the yeast Candida Albicans and skin issues.

Food Allergens

The majority of medical complaints, including skin problems, such as rosacea and seborrheic dermatitis, would be resolved when we eliminate the main allergens: wheat (gluten), dairy, peanuts, soy, yeast, eggs, and antibiotic-containing meats. Gluten is found in almost all processed foods. These allergens are the main source. There are the rare sensitivities to citrus fruits and bananas, but this is usually rare. I always recommend first eliminating the major allergens.

Over time, eating the highly allergenic foods, many individuals experience subtle increases in chronic inflammation, and irritation to the digestive tract. Forty percent of the population displays gluten intolerance. Gluten will affect the intestinal flora of a person who is sensitive to it.In addition to gluten in food, it's also found in some vitamin supplements, shampoos, and sunscreens.

While you might associate a food allergy with your face swelling up to the size of a basketball, it can manifest in other ways. Naturopathic physician Nicole Sundene, writing on her site Kitchen Table Medicine, explains that a food allergy can contribute to seborrheic dermatitis. Your body's rejection of the food can trigger the inflammation characteristic of this condition. She notes the most common offenders appear to be dairy, wheat and citrus fruits. Other common allergens include fish, such as bass, cod or flounder, shellfish such as crab, shrimp and lobster, peanuts, tree nuts and eggs. Experimenting with an elimination diet can help determine if certain foods worsen your symptoms. Cut out all suspected problem foods for a period of time and add them back one at a time to see which affect your condition. For specifics, work with doctor experienced in administering such diets.

Fight Allergens

Along with limiting specific foods, you want to make sure to include plenty of inflammation-fighting foods in your diet. Fruits and vegetables are rich sources of antioxidants, substances that can fight inflammation. When cooking, choose olive oil or canola oil over vegetable oils rich in omega-6 fatty acids. Eat more omega-3 fatty acids, found in cold-water fish such as salmon and tuna, flax seed, hemp seed and walnuts, provided you do not have any allergies to these items.

Borage Oil

Several studies have pointed out essential fatty acid (EFA) deficiency in individuals with atopic dermatitis. Researchers have hypothesized that a direct way to relieve symptoms may be to give dietary supplementation of GLA, concentrated in borage oil. Several studies have investigated the effect of borage oil supplementation on the symptoms and biochemistry associated with atopic dermatitis. One study reported significant and progressive improvement in itching, blistering, redness and oozing, with no change in dryness or scaling. The study also reported large, significant reductions in the need for antihistamines, steroid medications, and antibiotics for infections of skin lesions.

Caprylic Acid

Some have found caprylic acid to be helpful with bouts of seborrheic dermatitis. It is known to be antimicrobial, reducing systemic yeast overgrowth, which results in yeast infections of the skin. However, we need to look at the cause of the problem, which is almost always intestinal in nature.

Through research and observation, I have found those with suppressed immune systems are more susceptible to conditions such as seborrheic dermatitis. Those having previously taken doses of antibiotics are at greater risk since antibiotics kill both the good and bad intestinal bacteria. Yeast, Malassezia, which is a fungus, has been implicated in seborrheic dermatitis. Anti-fungal treatments have shown some temporary success in treatment but they are only curative and never eliminate the cause of the problem.

Food Tips

Certain foods in your daily diet might be the cause of your dandruff problem. From food allergies to nutritional deficiencies, there are many potential diet-related causes of dandruff. Some experts say that people who do not consume enough foods that contain zinc, B vitamins, and some types of fats are more prone to dandruff.

Foods That Help

- **Step Up Your Zinc Intake**: Clinical trials have shown zinc supplementation to be effective at controlling sebum production. Zinc requires vitamin B6 for proper absorption in the intestines, and is found in a variety of food like oysters, red meat, poultry, legumes, nuts, and grains.

- **Add Allicin to Your Diet**: Allicin is a potent health promoting compound found in garlic, onions and scallions, when these items are crushed or chopped. It has been shown to promote heart and cardiovascular health, prevent and treat cancer, and reduce high blood pressure, but it also helpful for people with dandruff due to its anti-fungal properties.

- **Eat Plenty of Foods Rich in B Vitamins**: If you are struggling with dandruff, eat plenty of foods rich in B vitamins. Evidence shows that B6 (pyridoxine) and B12 (riboflavin), can help reduce dandruff. It has been suggested that inefficient metabolism of carbohydrates and fatty acids could be one of the underlying causes of dandruff, and B-complex vitamins are known to play a crucial role in metabolic processes. Vitamin B6 can be found in a variety of foods like beans, meat, poultry, fish, and some fruits & vegetables.

Foods To Avoid

Reduce Sugar Consumption: A diet high in sugar that rapidly raises blood sugar levels can make dandruff worse in some people. Dandruff is often attributed to the Candida yeast, and sugary foods promote the overgrowth of this yeast in the body. Sugar also depletes the body of B vitamins, which are a key component of any anti-dandruff diet. A high intake of sugar also impacts the levels of antioxidant vitamins C and E in the body.

Stop Eating Dairy Products: Dairy products - including all milk products, milk, cheese, cottage cheese, yogurt, kefir, ice cream, etc. - are related to all kinds of diseases including cardiovascular diseases, autoimmune diseases, cancer, allergies, asthma, digestive diseases, thyroid problems, neurological diseases, etc. most people have lactose intolerance in some degree and this effects the skin immediately some people have Casein Sensitivity, The protein casein in dairy products creates serious problems just like the protein gluten in some grains like wheat. They can trigger an autoimmune response and/or mimic endorphins to cause changes in perception, mood, and behavior. The mechanism involved has to do with a failure of a particular enzyme which disassembles the gluten and casein protein, digestive process necessary for our bodies to extract the nutrients from these proteins. Because of the failure of this enzyme to do its job, a remaining undigested fragment of those proteins survive, and to our defense/immune system this fragment resembles a virus. Then, thinking that it is a virus, our bodies will trigger an immune/defense response to protect our bodies from the 'invader.' Because of this gluten or casein fragment is so similar to various disease-causing viruses, it will generate a complex reaction, an autoimmune response which is suspected to play a role in type I diabetes, multiple sclerosis, and autism. Complex immune responses damage different tissues in different people, so the range of diseases, is very diverse. Also, the undigested gluten or casein fragments look like opium-like drugs which can have a significant influence on our behavior and brains. They are literally drugs - and that is why people are so hooked on dairy and gluten!

Eliminate Food Allergens: What causes an allergic reaction in one person, however, may not cause a reaction in another. A elimination diet can be used to identify which foods worsen dandruff in an individual. This means removing any food or that is suspected of causing an allergy or intolerance from your diet for two to four weeks. If dandruff has disappeared or reduced significantly, the suspected foods and substances can be re-introduced to the diet, one food at a time. Systematically going through all the suspected allergens one by one, by consuming a suspect food or substance several times a day and then returning to the elimination diet for few days. If symptoms re-occur or worsen during this time, the person could be allergic to the food or chemical that was re-introduced.

<u>Chapter 3</u>

The Natural Way

Couse and Effect

Each year, about 70 percent of Americans are affected by some type of skin allergy. The most common allergens are poison ivy, poison oak and poison sumac. Other common substances that trigger skin allergies include construction materials used to build homes and offices, cleaning products, deodorants, cosmetics, and medications. Dermatitis of the earlobes can be caused by an allergy to earrings containing nickel. Chemicals in fragrances, skin creams and lotions, shampoos and shoes or clothing also can cause allergic reactions. Proper hygiene plays an important role in treatment. Frequent washing gets rid of the oils in the affected areas and diminishes symptoms. Sunlight inhibits the growth of the yeast; therefore exposure of affected areas to sun is helpful, although caution should be exercised to avoid sun damage.

A high level of toxicity in the body or an overactive immune system. An unhealthy diet and increased consumption of junk food, saturated fats, alcohol and sugars can cause an imbalance of nutrients in the body which in turn can cause a overgrowth of the yeast Candida albicans. This can then lead to an overactive immune system which produces histamine and eventually an eczema-like condition. As a result, the Candida yeast attacks the oil glands behind the ears, on the side of nose, scalp and chest.Stress and anxiety in adults can act as a catalyst in the manifestation of this condition.

Nutritional deficiencies in essential fatty acids, biotin (a B vitamin) and vitamin A - all of which are important for healthy skin. Biotin for example helps your body use essential fatty acids and assists in promoting healthy skin, hair, and nerves.The effect/overgrowth of a yeast organism Pityrosporum ovale, which normally resides in the hair follicles

Food intolerances most commonly to dairy products and gluten.

Apart from these main causes, there are other factors which are known to increase this condition. These include: genetic disposition, oily skin, obesity, Parkinson's disease, skin disorders such as acne, psoriasis and rosacea and AIDS which were mentioned in chapter 1 of this book.It is generally acknowledged that seborrheic dermatitis is caused by the internal malfunctioning of the body rather than any external factors.

Healthy Lifestyle

All Experts, Doctors, and Holistic practices, recommend a diet and lifestyle change to treat any problem especially skin disorders. Start by following this guideline :

Eat a healthy diet composed of 50-75% raw foods i.e. Plenty of raw fresh fruit and vegetables, including green leafy vegetables.

Some studies suggest a link between skin disorders, including eczema and psoriasis, and gluten allergy; therefore a gluten-free diet could be helpful.

Other foods to avoid are processed chocolate, dairy products, white flour, fried foods, seafood, nuts and anything containing sugar – even undiluted fruit juice which contains high levels of natural sugar.

Cutting down your intake of sugar, junk food and saturated fats and increasing your fiber intake can help reduce Candida infestation and clear the skin.

Increase your intake of essential fatty acids by eating more oily fish, seeds and nuts, and vitamin E which is found in avocado, nuts, seeds, cold-pressed oils, wheat germ and oatmeal. Both of these nutrients help your skin to keep its moisture intact and prevent dryness.

Do not eat any foods containing raw egg. Egg whites contain high levels of avidin, a protein which attaches to biotin and prevents it from being absorbed. Biotin is needed for healthy hair and skin. Mayonnaise and some types of ice cream contain raw egg.

Eat foods which are high in biotin such as liver, kidney, herrings, cooked eggs and some fruit and vegetables (sweetcorn, watermelon, cauliflower, tomatoes), especially dried mixed fruit.

Avoid smoking and drinking Alchohol- these can aggravate skin conditions and inhibit the treatment measures.

Many nutritionists recommend a fasting program once a month to improve this condition; you should look for professional consultation on this matter.

Wear clothes made of natural fibers that allow the skin to breath. Avoid tight clothing.

Exercise regularly it will keep the mind fresh and the body active and help eliminate toxins and purify your body and your skin.

Relaxation and plentiful sleep are so important. Ensure that you take steps to relax by practising yoga or meditation for example. Do not underestimate the effect of the mind on the health of the body. Stress has a negative impact on the whole body including the digestive system and the skin, and can cause inflammation to occur.

Avoid chemical-based and pharmacy products which are likely to worsen your condition. If they contain synthetic chemicals and mineral oils, the ingredients can provoke a response in the skin or make the skin drier. Switching to a natural or certified organic product for sensitive skin could make a significant difference.

includes burdock and sarsaparilla, nettle and antioxidants such as lycopene, Vitaflavan, vitamin A, and zinc with Dandelion, rutin, folic acid and vitamin B6 to help maintain healthy skin.

Conventional Treatment

Conventional treatments are topical and do not deal with the internal causes of the condition. These include salicylic acid bath, selenium sulfide, and coal tar soaps. Steroid solutions are also used however over usage of steroids has known side-effects and can also increase the resistance of disease-causing organisms. These treatments can all worsen seborrhea because they contain chemicals which may irritate the skin.

Chapter 4

Skin Treatment

Skin Diagnosis

Dermatitis is a clinical diagnosis based on the location and appearance of lesions. In infants, it may present as thick white or yellow greasy scales on the scalp. In adolescents and adults, seborrheic dermatitis typically presents as flaky, greasy, erythematous patches on the scalp, nasolabial folds, ears, eyebrows, anterior chest, or upper back.

The differential diagnosis is lengthy, but the correct diagnosis can usually be made clinically by the characteristic distribution of lesions and varying course of the disease. If the diagnosis is uncertain, a biopsy can confirm the presence of seborrheic dermatitis. The diagnosis can be challenging in patients with darker skin, but the same principles apply.

Pathophysiology

Although the pathophysiology of seborrheic dermatitis is not completely understood, the mechanisms of effective therapies coupled with results of recent biomolecular studies provide clues about the causes. The redness, itching, and scaling associated with seborrheic dermatitis are caused by changes in skin cell functioning. Malassezia yeast seems to cause a nonspecific immune response that begin the cascade of skin changes that occur in seborrheic dermatitis. Malassezia is a normal component of skin flora, but in persons with seborrheic dermatitis, the yeast invade the stratum corneum, releasing lipases that result in free fatty acid formation and cause the inflammatory process to begin. Malassezia thrive in high-lipid environments, so the presence of free fatty acids enhances the growth of the yeast. The inflammation causes stratum corneum hyperproliferation (scaling) and incomplete corneocyte differentiation, which alters the stratum corneum barrier and impairs its function; thus increasing access for Malassezia and allowing water to more readily leave the cells.

Based on the current understanding of the pathophysiology of the condition, the treatments for seborrheic dermatitis make biologic sense. Keratolytics (sulfur and salicylic acid) help remove the outer layers of the hyperproliferating stratum corneum. Coal tar is thought to decrease the rate of stratum corneum production. Antifungals decrease the Malassezia population, whereas antiinflammatories such as corticosteroids and calcineurin inhibitors decrease the inflammatory response. Many of the current treatments for seborrheic dermatitis have multiple effects (antifungal, anti-inflammatory, regulation of stratum corneum production), thereby combatting the skin changes on multiple levels. The severity of symptoms can be affected by stress and sun exposure, and often has a variable course despite treatment.

Natural Products

The treatment of infantile and adolescents seborrheic dermatitis consist primarily of using pure organic skin products and natural shampoos with no S.L.S and using emollients that help loosen scales like natural and organic oils, for example, olive and almond oils. Scales can then be removed by rubbing with a cloth or infant hair brush.

There are no shampoos that have been approved by the U.S. Food and Drug inistration for treatment of seborrheic dermatitis in children younger than two years. Treatment of seborrheic dermatitis in adolescents is identical to that in adults; the primary goals are to lessen the visible signs of the condition and to reduce pruritus and erythema. Treatment includes over-the-counter shampoos and topical antifungals, calcineurin inhibitors, and corticosteroids. Because of seborrheic dermatitis is a chronic condition, ongoing maintenance therapy is often necessary, so going as natural as possible is the only way to control our skin problems.

Over-the counter dandruff shampoos containing sodium and S.L.S can work for a while but will stop preventing dandruff after some time. So it's important to use clean shampoos with has much fewer chemicals as possible. Look for natural shampoos with nettle and Tea tree that are proved to help scalp problems. When your diet is good, and you use clean products your skin will soon feel the difference and will get better.

For soothing the skin use natural oils and creams that will hydrate the skin and help the skin to heal and reduce irritation. You can find many recipes in the complimentary book they are all safe to use with skin disorders as they are pure and contribute to the natural breathing process of the skin. When the problem persists, you can incorporate professional products that have effective ingredients to treat your problem. You can find the right product for your skin disorder on my site www.laorcare.com

Alpha/Beta Hydroxy Acids

Alpha hydroxy acids are a group of natural acids found in foods. Alpha hydroxy acids include citric acid (found in citrus fruits), glycolic acid (found in sugar cane), lactic acid (found in sour milk), malic acid (found in apples), tartaric acid (found in grapes), and others.While alpha hydroxy acids are soluble only in water, beta hydroxy acid is soluble in oil. Salicylic acid is the only beta hydroxy acid present on the planet. This means that beta hydroxy acid is better for oily skin with whiteheads and blackheads, while alpha hydroxy acids are for thickened, photo-damaged skin that is not prone to breakouts.

According to experts, products rich in AHAs contribute positively to smoother and clearer skin. Chemically, these acids are a series of compounds that are made from well-known food products. Few examples of these acids, which are most widely used, include glycolic acid made from sugar cane, citric acid made from citrus fruits, lactic acid from sour milk, and malic acid extracted from apples.

Interestingly, these acids have a long history for their use for younger-looking skin. This history traces back to ancient Egyptians who used this natural compounds widely. Today, their popularity has shot up like a missile. Present in many facial creams and peels and in several skin care products after approval by FDA, AHAs have become vital ingredients in several creams, shampoos, lightening lotions, seborrheic dermatitis and acne moisturizers.

These acids mainly work as exfoliants. They break the bond between the cells and epidermis so that the dead skin cells are dismissed. This makes space for growth of new skin. Apart from exfoliators, alpha hydroxy acids can even boost or kindle the production of elastin and collagen. Moreover, these acids help cleansing the skin by lightening the appearance of wrinkles, dryness, blotchy pigmentation due to sun, and roughness. However, this is only possible if the acid is used consistently and constantly for a few month. According to experts, alpha hydroxy acids act as ideal exfoliators, blood circulation boosters, fine line and wrinkle reducers, dark spot lighteners, and blackheads and Rosacea, seborrheic dermatitisacne fighters.

Although there are so many reasons of using an AHA skin care product, there are some limitations to bear as well. If you are using products to be used at home with low concentrations of acid, it might take months to heal your skin, so always choose professional products with the right concentration and pH level for your problem.

Products available at over the counter have alpha hydroxy acids that are usually safe for a majority of people. However, they might be unsuitable for those having sensitive skin, A seborrheic dermatitis, and rosacea due to increased risk of rash. In this case, this people need to look for a product that are with no chemicals and mineral oils and were carefully designed to treat this problem with safe concentration. Usually, over-the-counter AHA products like lotions and moisturizers have not even 5% of glycolic acid, while cosmeceuticals of medical-grade tend to contain 8 to 14%.

Retinoids and Azelaic Acid - This best combination of ingredients are good in low concentration for Rosacea and sensitive skin. Retinoid is derived from vitamin A. You apply this medication in the evening, beginning with three times a week, then daily as your skin becomes used to it. It works better if it's combined with Azelaic Acid in the product or a separate product, the Azelaic acid works on the inflammation.

Retinoid Acid - Vitamin A is used as an ingredient in certain medicines. Vitamin A is found very useful to treat non-inflammatory types of Rosacea on face. It can open clogged pores, Retinoids reduce the excess production of skin oil. For sensitive skin, it is best to use Retinoids up to 1%.

Azelaic Acid - Azelaic acid is a natural chemical that's produced by the action of a particular yeast. It is a naturally occurring acid that may be found in grains like wheat. This chemical has three main and very distinct properties that have elevated its role in Rosacea treatment: The ability to fight off anaerobic bacteria that cause the pustules and lesions on the face, back, neck and chest. The ability to reducing inflammation. Using 5% Azelaic Acid for Sensitive skin is safe.

Tea tree oil - kills the bacteria and is very antiseptic, so it helps the skin heal and keeps it pure and protected from bacteria.

Clay Masks to Purify the Skin - One product which always gives best results is the clay mask. Clay is good to help to reduce oil levels. It can eventually lead to drastic reduction in the number of new breakouts.

Sun Protection - Look for sunscreens that are fragrance free, Mineral Oil, and Parabens free and use ingredients such as zinc oxide or titanium dioxide as these tend to be less irritating. Check the labels and try different products. Consult with your dermatologist if you continue to have trouble finding a suitable product. All infants should be kept out of direct sun and be covered by protective clothing when possible. If sun exposure is unavoidable, sunscreen should be applied to exposed areas. Sunscreens have been deemed safe for infants older than 6 months of age. Choose a broad spectrum sunscreen with an SPF 30 or higher but not more than 50 SPF that can contain harmful chemicals. The protective ability of sunscreen is rated by its Sun Protection Factor (SPF) – the higher the SPF, the stronger the protection. Sunscreens labeled as "broad spectrum" indicate that they have passed the test for protection against UVA. Spread sunscreen evenly over all uncovered skin, including ears, and lips, but avoid the eyelids.Wear sunscreen year round whenever you are outside.Do not use sun lamps, tanning beds, or tanning salons they are all bad for Rosacea and seborrheic dermatitis problems.

Chapter 5

Balance Is The Key

Hormones Control

Hormones have profound effects on your mental, physical and emotional health and in some people can create skin disorders. These chemical messengers play a major role in controlling your appetite, weight and mood, among other things. Normally, your endocrine glands produce the precise amount of each hormone needed for various processes in your body. However, hormonal imbalances have become increasingly common with today's fast-paced modern lifestyle. In addition, certain hormones decline with age, and some people experience more dramatic decrease than others. Fortunately, a nutritious diet and other healthy lifestyle behaviors may help improve your hormonal health, allow you to feel and perform your best and make your skin healthy again.

Balanced Tips

Here are some Ways To Balance Your Hormones easy and fast:

1. Engage in Regular Exercise - Physical activity can strongly influence hormonal health. A major benefit of exercise is its ability to reduce insulin levels and increase insulin sensitivity. Insulin is a hormone that has several functions. One is allowing cells to take up sugar and amino acids from the bloodstream, which are then used for energy and maintaining muscle. However, a little insulin goes a long way. Too much can be downright dangerous. High insulin levels have been linked to inflammation, heart disease, diabetes and cancer. What's more, they are connected to insulin resistance, a condition in which your cells don't respond properly to insulin's signals.Many types of physical activity have been found to increase insulin sensitivity and reduce insulin levels, including aerobic exercise, strength training and endurance exercise. In a 24-week study of obese women, exercise increased participants' insulin sensitivity and levels of adiponectin, a hormone that has anti-inflammatory effects and helps regulate metabolism.Being physically active may also help boost levels of muscle-maintaining hormones that decline with age, such as testosterone, IGF-1, DHEA and growth hormone. For people who are unable to perform vigorous exercise, even regular walking may increase these hormone levels, potentially improving strength and quality of life. Although a combination of resistance and aerobic training seems to provide the best results, engaging in any type of physical activity on a regular basis is beneficial.

Summary: Performing strength training, aerobics, walking or other forms of physical activity can modify hormone levels in a way that reduces the risk of disease and protects muscle mass during the aging process.

2. Eat Enough Protein at Every Meal - Consuming an adequate amount of protein is extremely important. Dietary protein provides essential amino acids that your body can't make on its own and must be consumed every day in order to maintain muscle, bone, and skin health.

In addition, protein influences the release of hormones that control appetite and food intake. Research has shown that eating protein decreases levels of the "hunger hormone" ghrelin and stimulates the production of hormones that help you feel full, including PYY and GLP-1. In one study, men produced 20% more GLP-1 and 14% more PYY after eating a high-protein meal than after eating a meal that contained a normal amount of protein. What's more, participants' hunger ratings decreased by 25% more after the high-protein meal compared to the normal-protein meal. In another study, women who consumed a diet containing 30% protein experienced an increase in GLP-1 and greater feelings of fullness than when they ate a diet containing 10% protein.

What's more, they experienced a increase in metabolism and fat burning. To optimize hormone health, experts recommend consuming a minimum of 20–30 grams of protein per meal from vegetarian or animal source.

3. Avoid Sugar and Refined Carbs - Sugar and refined carbs have been linked to a number of health problems. Indeed, avoiding or minimizing these foods may be instrumental in optimizing hormone function and avoiding obesity, diabetes and other diseases. Studies have consistently shown that fructose can increase insulin levels and promote insulin resistance, especially in overweight and obese people with prediabetes or diabetes. Importantly, fructose makes up at least half of most types of sugar. This includes natural forms like honey and maple syrup, besides, to high-fructose corn syrup and refined table sugar.

In one study, people with pre-diabetes experienced similar increases in insulin levels and insulin resistance whether they consumed 1.8 ounces (50 grams) of honey, sugar or high-fructose corn syrup. In addition, diets high in refined carbs like white bread and pretzels may promote insulin resistance in a large portion of adults and adolescents. By contrast, following a low- or moderate-carb diet based on whole foods may reduce insulin levels in overweight and obese people with prediabetes and other insulin-resistant conditions like polycystic ovary syndrome (PCOS).

Summary: Diets high in sugar and refined carbs have been shown to drive insulin resistance. Avoiding these foods and reducing overall carb intake may decrease insulin levels and increase insulin sensitivity

4. Learn to Manage Stress - Stress can increase your hormones production. Two major hormones affected by stress are cortisol and adrenaline, which is also called pinephrine. Cortisol is known as "the stress hormone" because it helps your body cope with stress over the long term. Adrenaline is the "fight-or-flight" hormone that provides your body with a surge of energy to respond to immediate danger. However, unlike hundreds of years ago when these hormones were mainly triggered by threats from predators, today they're usually triggered by people's busy, often overwhelming lifestyles. Unfortunately, chronic stress causes cortisol levels to remain elevated, which can lead to excessive calorie intake and obesity, including increased belly fat.

Elevated adrenaline levels can cause high blood pressure, rapid heart rate and anxiety. However, these symptoms are usually fairly short-lived because, unlike cortisol, adrenaline is less likely to become chronically elevated. Research has shown that you may be able to lower your cortisol levels by engaging in stress-reducing techniques like meditation, yoga, massage and listening to relaxing music. A review of studies found that massage therapy not only reduced cortisol levels by an average of 31%, but also increased levels of the mood-boosting hormone serotonin by 28% and dopamine by 31%, on average. Try to devote yourself at least 10–15 minutes per day to stress-reducing activities like meditation, even if you don't feel you have the time.

Summary: Engaging in stress-reduction behaviors like meditation, yoga, massage and listening to soothing music can help normalize your levels of the stress hormone cortisol.

5. Consume Healthy Fats - Including high-quality natural fats in your diet may help reduce insulin resistance and appetite. Medium-chain triglycerides (MCTs) are unique fats that are taken up directly by the liver for immediate use as energy. They have been shown to reduce insulin resistance in overweight and obese people, as well as in people with diabetes. MCTs are found in coconut oil, palm oil, and pure MCT oil.

Dairy fats and monounsaturated fat in olive oil and nuts also seem to increase insulin sensitivity, based on studies in healthy adults and those with diabetes, prediabetes, fatty liver and elevated triglycerides. Additionally studies have shown that consuming healthy fat at meals triggers the release of hormones that help you feel full and satisfied, including GLP-1, PYY and cholecystokinin (CCK). On the other hand, trans fats have been found to promote insulin resistance and increase the storage of belly fat. To optimize hormone health, consume a healthy fat source at each meal.

Summary: Including healthy natural fats in your diet and avoiding unhealthy trans fats can help reduce insulin resistance and stimulate the production of hormones that help control appetite.

6. Drink Green Tea - Green tea is one of the healthiest beverages around. In addition to metabolism-boosting caffeine, it contains a antioxidant known as epigallocatechin gallate (EGCG), which has been credited with several health benefits. Research suggests that consuming green tea may increase insulin sensitivity and lower insulin levels in both healthy people and those with insulin-resistant conditions like obesity and diabetes. In one detailed analysis of 17 studies, the highest-quality studies linked green tea to significantly lower fasting insulin levels. A few controlled studies found that green tea didn't seem to reduce insulin resistance or insulin levels when compared to a placebo. However, these results may have been due to individual responses.

Since green tea has other health benefits and most studies suggest that it may provide some improvement in insulin response, you may want to consider drinking one to three cups per day.

Summary: Green tea has been linked to increased insulin sensitivity and lower insulin levels for people who are overweight, obese or have diabetes.

7. Eat Fatty Fish oil Often - Fatty fish is by far the best source of long-chain omega-3 fatty acids, which have impressive anti-inflammatory properties. Research suggests they may also have beneficial effects on hormonal health, including reducing levels of the stress hormones cortisol and adrenaline. A small study observed the effect of consuming omega-3 fats on men's performance on a mental stress test. The study found that after men consumed a diet rich in omega-3 fats for three weeks, they experienced significantly smaller increases in cortisol and epinephrine during the test than when they followed their regular diet. Besides, some studies have found that increasing your intake of long-chain omega-3 fatty acids may reduce insulin resistance related to obesity, polycystic ovary syndrome and gestational diabetes. Gestational diabetes occurs during pregnancy in women who did not have diabetes prior to becoming pregnant. Like type 2 diabetes, it is characterized by insulin resistance and elevated blood sugar levels. In one study, women with gestational diabetes took 1,000 mg of omega-3 fatty acids daily for six weeks.

The omega-3 group experienced significant reductions in insulin levels, insulin resistance and the inflammatory marker C-reactive protein (CRP) compared to women who received a placebo. For optimal health, include two or more servings per week of fatty fish like salmon, sardines, herring and mackerel.

Summary: Long-chain omega-3 fatty acids may help lower cortisol and epinephrine, increase insulin sensitivity and decrease insulin levels in obese and insulin-resistant individuals.

8. Get Consistent, High-Quality Sleep - No matter how nutritious your diet is and how much exercise you get, your health will suffer if you don't get enough restorative sleep. Poor sleep has been linked to imbalances of many hormones, including insulin, cortisol, leptin, ghrelin and growth hormone. In one study of men whose sleep was restricted to five hours per night for one week, insulin sensitivity decreased by 20%, on average. Another study looked at the effects of sleep restriction on healthy young men. When their sleep was restricted for two days, their leptin declined by 18%, their ghrelin increased by 28% and their hunger increased by 24%. In addition, the men craved high-calorie, high-carb foods. Moreover, it's not only the quantity of sleep you get that matters. Quality of sleep is also important.

Your brain needs uninterrupted sleep that allows it to go through all five stages of each sleep cycle. This is especially important for the release of growth hormone, which occurs mainly at night during deep sleep. To maintain optimal hormonal balance, aim for at least seven hours of high-quality sleep per night.

Summary: Inadequate or poor-quality sleep has been shown to decrease fullness hormones, increase hunger and stress hormones, reduce growth hormone and increase insulin resistance.

9. Eat Eggs Anytime - Eggs are one of the most nutritious foods on the planet. They've been shown to beneficially affect hormones that regulate food intake, including lowering levels of insulin and ghrelin, and increasing PYY. In one study, men had lower ghrelin and insulin levels after eating eggs at breakfast than after eating a bagel for breakfast. What's more, they felt fuller and ate fewer calories over the next 24 hours after eating the eggs. Importantly, these positive effects on hormones seem to occur when people eat both the egg yolk and egg white. For instance, another study found that eating whole eggs as part of a low-carb diet increased insulin sensitivity and improved several heart health markers more than a low-carb diet that included only egg whites.

Most studies have looked at the effects of eating eggs at breakfast because that is when people typically consume them. However, these nutrition powerhouses can be eaten at any meal, and hard-boiled eggs make a great portable snack.

Summary: Eggs are extremely nutritious and may help reduce insulin resistance, suppress your appetite and make you feel full.

10. Consume a High-Fiber Diet - Fiber, especially the soluble type, is an important component of a healthy diet. Studies have found that it increases insulin sensitivity and stimulates the production of hormones that make you feel full and satisfied. Although soluble fiber tends to produce the strongest effects on appetite and eating, insoluble fiber may also play a role. One study in overweight and obese people found that consuming a type of soluble fiber called oligofructose increased PYY levels, and consuming the insoluble fiber cellulose tended to increase GLP-1 levels. Both types of fiber caused a reduction in appetite. To protect against insulin resistance and overeating, make sure you eat fiber-rich foods on a daily basis.

Summary: High fiber intake has been linked to improvements in insulin sensitivity and the hormones that control hunger, fullness and food intake.

11. Avoid Overeating and Undereating - Eating too much or too little may result in hormonal shifts that lead to weight problems. Overeating is shown to increase insulin levels and reduce insulin sensitivity, especially in overweight and obese people who are insulin resistant. In one study, insulin-resistant obese adults who ate a 1,300-calorie meal experienced nearly twice the increase in insulin as lean people and "metabolically healthy" obese people who consumed an identical meal. On the other hand, cutting your calorie intake too much can increase levels of the stress hormone cortisol, which is known to promote weight gain when it's elevated. One study found that restricting food intake to less than 1,200 calories per day led to increased cortisol levels. Interestingly, a study from 1996 even suggests that very low-calorie diets could potentially trigger insulin resistance in some people, an effect you might expect to see in people with diabetes. Eating within your own personal calorie range can help you maintain hormonal balance and a healthy weight.

Summary: Consuming too many or too few calories can lead to hormonal imbalances. Aim to eat at least 1,200 calories per day for optimal health.

12. Stay Away From Sugary Beverages - Sugar in any form is unhealthy. However, liquid sugars appear to be the worst by far. Studies suggest large amounts of sugar-sweetened beverages may contribute to insulin resistance, especially in overweight and obese adults and children. In one study, when overweight people consumed 25% of their calories in the form of high-fructose beverages, they experienced higher blood insulin levels, a reduction in insulin sensitivity and increased belly fat storage. Additionally, research has shown that drinking sugary beverages leads to excessive calorie intake because it doesn't trigger the same fullness signals that eating solid foods does. Avoiding sugar-sweetened beverages may be one of the best things you can do to improve your hormone balance.

Summary: High intake of sugary beverages has consistently been linked to higher insulin levels and insulin resistance in overweight and obese adults and children.

The Bottom Line

Your hormones are involved in the every aspect of your health including the health of your skin. You need them in very specific amounts for your body to function optimally.Hormonal imbalances may increase your risk of obesity, diabetes, heart disease and other health problems. Despite the fact that aging and other factors are beyond your control, there are many steps you can take to help your hormones function optimally. Consuming nutritious foods, exercising on a regular basis and engaging in other healthy behaviors can go a long way toward improving your hormonal health.

Chapter 6

Home Remedies

Just Natural

If you are fighting Rosacea, seborrheic dermatitis or dandruff and have already browsed around online previous to reading this, you will know that many people claim to have found an effective home remedy for seborrheic dermatitis on the scalp. Some of these methods might in fact work, while others are just sheer pushes to get you to purchase some type of herbal product or natural cream. The best way to find proved home remedies for seborrheic dermatitis on the scalp is to collect data. In this chapter we will do exactly that. In this chapter, you will find a summarized overview of home remedies that have worked for others. The remedies are listed in order of popularity and how significant the results have been for me. Please keep in mind that most people believe seborrheic dermatitis to be a fungus/yeast issue. For this reason when you look at the most common home remedies for seborrheic dermatitis you will notice that most act as anti-fungals, aimed at destroying these skin invading organisms. You can find more recipes to treat your skin in my complimentary ebook " Natural Beauty Recipes" you can download for free.

You can download my free Recipe Book that includes all the products you need that are safe for you to use. Here are more natural ways to treat Rosacea, seborrheic dermatitis and dandruff:

Honey and Water Treatment

This is my personal favorite. The treatment is, however, fairly difficult due to the stickiness of honey. Basically all you have to do is apply honey water to the affected areas and everything around them for 3 hours (leaving it on). Once the +3 hours are up you simply wash the honey off and go about business as usual.

To make your honey water all you do is mix 4 parts honey to 1 part boiled water. The boiled water part is very important. Personally I found that rinsing the honey with boiled water after treatment also works much better than regular tap water.

The honey is said to work by being an anti-fungal and anti-bacterial agent. This effect kills of the microbes causing the seborrheic dermatitis and dandruff in the first place. Another positive effect of honey is that draws moisture in to the skin and locks it in, helping to keep the skin supple.

Coconut Oil Treatment

A very popular treatment is coconut oil applied for a few hours onto the affected skin. Best results are said to occur if a show cap is worn. The coconut oil loosens the scale brought about by seborrheic dermatitis and fights the fungus which causes it.

To use coconut oil, you basically take an amount which you estimate to cover all of the affected skin (typically about 1/2 a teaspoon). You then rub the solid coconut oil between your hands until it liquefies. Then you careful massage the oil into the skin making sure to stimulate the pores. Once applied you can optionally wrap your head in a shower cap or towel (the locked in heat helps the oil stay liquid).

The fungus fighting activity is speculated to come from coconuts oil unique fatty acid profile. It has two fungus destroying fatty acids in its arsenal. One being Lauric Acid and the other Caprylic Acid. Together they form quite a powerful duo and help stop seborrheic dermatitis in its tracks.

Apple Cider Vinegar Treatment

Another extremely popular seborrheic dermatitis is apple cider vinegar. With a long history in skin scare treatment this is a true powerhouse. The strong acidity of the main acid (malic acid) found in apple cider vinegar help destroy seborrheic dermatitis causing fungus and restore the skins natural acidic environment.

The most recommended method of using apple cider vinegar is in a 50/50 ratio with water. Once again most people recommend the water used to be either boiled or bottled. Mix the apple cider vinegar together with the water in a small container and apply to the affected skin in the shower.

Leave this solution on the skin and let it absorb for as long as possible (roughly 10-15 minutes while you shower). You will likely feel a stingy sensation if the skin is badly damaged. If this is the case I recommend quickly rinsing off and applying a more diluted solution (75/25). Once you get out of the shower and dry off the vinegar smell should quickly fade (roughly 30 minutes to an hour depending on hair length).

Apple cider vinegar is made up mainly of malic acid. This unique acid is very powerful against different types of fungus and yeast. It has also been made very popular due to a rising popularity anti-yeast diets such as the candida diet and the rising number of women caught with yeast infections. Not only is apple cider vinegar good when applied topically, but it has a long history of internal use. Many people swear by its benefits and consume it every single day on an empty stomach or with food.

Baking Soda Treatment

Baking soda has a long history of successfully fighting fungus. Many people online have had great success with it and it is also much less of a hassle to use then other methods listed here. This is mainly due to its lack of smell and quick treatment time.

Mix half a tea spoon of luring baking soda with half a cup of water. Apply this solution to the affected skin for 5 to 10 minutes. After the baking soda has had time to do its work, simply rinse off with cool water.

As an extra bonus you can follow up with a quick rinse of apple cider vinegar diluted with water (as used in treatment above). This will quickly restore the skin natural acidic state and help keep it protected.

Baking soda works in the opposite way of apple cider vinegar. Instead of using acid to fight the fungus the alkalinity of the baking soda is used. Fungus will quickly die and breakdown if the environment is too alkaline and this is exactly what the baking soda does.

Tea Tree Oil Shampoo

A remedy used in lots of skin care products due to its anti-bacterial and anti-fungal properties tea tree oil has had a sharp increase in popular in recent years. However, when it comes to remedying seborrheic dermatitis the results are quite mixed. It works fabulously for some while not actually makes things works for others. Feel free to give it a try, but be sure to closely monitor how your skin reacts and adjust treatment as necessary.

How to Use Tea Tree Oil to Remedy Seborrheic Dermatitis

With tea tree oil you have quite a large number of options. Basically, they fall into two categories:

Pre-Made Tea Tree Oil Remedies - If you go for the pre-made approach simply hit your nearest supermarket and look for any shampoo that contains tea tree oil. Try to go for the ones that have the least ingredients and clear from SLS, Parabens, and salts.

Home Made Tea Tree Oil Remedy - If you want to know exactly what goes on your skin an custom solution is for you. Tea tree oil is safe not diluted but sometimes strong if used on its own, The most popular method of using it topically is to mix it with a carrier oil such as olive, sesame seed, or coconut oil. Out of the these three oils, I highly recommend either sesame seed oil or coconut oil as many other oils tend to actually promote the growth of the seborrheic dermatitis causing fungus.

When mixing you typically only need 4-5 drops of tea tree oil per teaspoon of the carrier oil. However, even this can irritate very sensitive skin. To see what works for you, try this concentration on a small patch of seborrheic dermatitis effected skin and observe for irritation. If all is well go ahead and apply it all the effected skin and leave on for 30-60 minutes. Once it has had time to soak in rinse off with cool water and wash regularly.

Tea tree oil is a well known anti-microbial and anti-fungal agent. When applied topically and left to soak-in, the tea tree oil goes to work combating the seborrheic dermatitis fungus. If the tea tree oil does it job and destroys enough of the fungus, you will likely see great improvements in the seborrheic dermatitis.

CONCLUSION

Bringing the balance to our lives will restore balance in the face, working on our self-esteem will help us overcome Acne. The food is a crucial element in healing the Acne mainly milk products, Gluten, and Simple Sugars. Keep eating junk food won't help for anything.

SD is a common skin condition seen frequently in clinical practice. Despite its frequency, much controversy remains regarding its pathogenesis. This controversy extends to its classification in the spectrum of cutaneous diseases, having been classified as a form of dermatitis, or a fungal disease, or a disease closely related with psoriasis.

Take good care of the face with quality products and treat the scars with a Roller. Acne that comes from genetics can be beaten with good mind healthy foods and by taking good care of our faces with efficient products.

For Example Seborrhea home care treatment by LAOR – day and night treatment

Laor Skin Care Series act to balance the sebaceous glands in the face and reduce the production of sebum secreted by the skin, this action reduces skin redness and scaling that accompanies it. Amino acids, oils and vitamins are the most effective ingredients treating the Seborrhea problem. We also recommend that those who suffer from this skin disorder will use only natural shampoo and soap to stop irritate the skin and slow down the production of sebum in the skin. We recommend regular use of the products morning and night to keep the balance of the sebaceous glands and thus reduce the problem of visible seborrhea.

Day Care – starts with a thorough cleansing of the skin with hydrophilic soap, product number 1 or peeling number 8. Then use cream No 21 / -21 that contain AHA and BHA. This creams balances and reduces sebaceous secretions that cause scaly skin and redness. The daily treatment should be completed with moisture serum No 41 or moisture cream No52. It is important to put on a sun protection cream, product number 72 to reduce the stimulation of sebaceous glands from sun and pollution.

Night Care – includes the removal of dead cells and dirt that has accumulated on the skin during the day, Product No 8. and in-depth of the skin treating sebaceous glands with creams containing amino acids especially Retinol cream No 22 / -22, that balances the secretion of sebum and helps to peel of dead cells that block the normal action of breathing in the skin system, causing skin discomfort expressed in dryness and redness. For best calming results, it is recommended to use serum No 42 to ease any discomfort of the skin and give it anti-aging properties.

It is essential to repeat here that before you launch into any of this top acne treatments, consult a physician or a skin specialist. It will ensure that you choose the right treatment depending on the type of acne you are suffering from, the type of skin you have and the severity of the problem.

Remember, Rosacea is a preventable, controllable and treatable skin condition as long as you commit to proper care and continuous self-improvement. Instead of getting stressed by the situation, take the initiative and improve your health, your diet, your lifestyle and your self-esteem.

In conclusion, just remember that combination skin rosacea treatments are the best options if you have combination skin. Products that are designed either for oily or dry skin generally will not produce the most hoped-for results. Yes, treating combination skin rosacea is probably twice as hard, but with perseverance, implementing a regular skin care routine, using appropriate products, a person can eventually get rid of acne.

Thank you very much for reading the book. If you loved the book, I would appreciate it if you can write a review of the book for me. If you have any question about the book feel free to contact me at orilaor@outlook.com.

For 20$ Coupon for www.laorcare.com were you can find all the professional products to clear your Acne and scars, send the word: LOVEISTHEKEY to my mail.

With sincere love Ori Laor